THIS NOTEBOOK BELONGS TO:

www.ingramcontent.com/pod-product-compliance
Lightning Source LLC
Chambersburg PA
CBHW020326290526
45785CB00007B/2932